God Still Loves Aging Beauties

God Still Loves Aging Beauties

C.K.Inniss

Contents

- *About the author* -

Feast of the Lord Transformation Ministries
Evangelist Dr. Cynthia (Cki) Inniss

Evangelist Cki was born in Rome, Georgia to George and Vera Kinnebrew. Like most of God's children, there were many prodigal years where she sought what the world had to offer, finding ridicule, heartache and disappointments too numerous to relate here. After high school and a brief career foray into nursing, attending Floyd School of Nursing, Mount Berry College where she was capped, She joined the military and served her country for eight years.

While in the military she met and married her husband of 29 years, Evangelist Marco Aurelio Inniss, at that time a military officer. Through this union she traveled extensively throughout Europe living in Germany for three years, Spain for four years, and a subsequent three years in the Republic of Panama, where she earned a Bachelor's degree in Business. A 10-year career with the Federal Government in Washington, D.C., followed; where she achieved the GS-13 level as a Logistics Manager.

Germany was a pivotal time in her life as she conceived and gave birth to a daughter there in 1976, Kimara Jestina Inniss, who is now married to her son-in-law, Raymond Graves. Kimara and Raymond are both ordained ministers serving Christ with their whole hearts!

It was in Spain that she met Jesus again, this time as an adult, giving her heart and life to Him. The seed of salvation was firmly planted many years ago in a Rome,

Georgia church called Mt. Sinai CME church, where her mother, a devout and Holy Ghost filled woman of God, insisted her children go often! Since that time of rebirth in Spain, she has attended "The School of the Holy Spirit," for the past 25 years.

Also in Spain, she met Reverend Gloria Cherry (a divine connection), who has become her mother in the ministry and life-long friend! In 2001, Pastor Cherry, an anointed healing minister who pastors Healing Wings Christian Center in Dover, Delaware, and travels extensively to provide healing crusades, ordained Evangelist Inniss to preach and teach this great gospel of the kingdom! To God belongs all the glory for the great things He has done!

DEDICATION

I dedicate this labor of love to all women and even to any man who is spiritually "man enough" to embrace this truth in support of your woman! Many times men also have a tendency towards erratic behavior when confronted with age, there's wisdom herein for you as well! It is my hope that the Holy Spirit of God who breathed this message through me to you, will anoint your eyes, ears and heart to see, hear and hold onto this message. My hope is that you will be wholly released from demonic suggestions concerning beauty that threaten to conquer the soul.

As we expose the lies of the devil concerning beauty, and unfold the wisdom of God concerning your true beauty (resident beneath your skin), you'll begin to stand up tall and straight, and never again relegate yourself to the cellar of God's blessings! This word from God will change your life! Jesus placed Satan and all his lies and distortions under His feet *and* under your feet. Don't let the enemy steal even one more minute of your peace!

"If the Son therefore shall make you free, ye shall be free indeed!"
-John 8:36-

Foreword

Soul, why art thou cast down, why art thou disquieted in me? Dreaming unfulfilled dreams year after year after year can cause the soul to writhe in turmoil and pain. Maybe as a child you either believed yourself to be beautiful and expected positive attention from the world, or perhaps you were so unattractive you never really expected that anything good would come to you. Maybe you grew up the middle child in a family of five children and believed silently you were a mistake, unwanted by your parents. No matter the reason for the turmoil, as the years progress your soul is continually disquieted.

A girl child who lacks nourishment during the crucial growth process will experience what we call "stunted growth." A young woman who longs for words of affirmation from the man in her life (her father), and never receives them, can become what I call a compliment junky. You're starved for affection-won't somebody please tell me I'm pretty and worthwhile! Then one day a man walks into your life and tells you you're pretty (any old man), and you're off to the races. Each man that deigns to ply you with compliments from that day forward is rewarded with your undying affection and gift giving. It's like riding a perpetual roller coaster to hell! You've sold yourself short, given away your most priceless possession to men who regard you the same as they regard their old sneakers: once they're used, they are good only to be cast out!

One day a real man shows up and sweeps you off your feet with the marital broom of forever. But, you still cannot accept this largess for what it truly represents (can't forgive yourself for giving away your treasure). How can he love you with the kind of love that only blushing brides receive? Doesn't he see beneath the surface of the make-up plaster and fake hair, to the depths of your soul where there is spiritual bankruptcy? On your wedding day you blush because of the secret you hide deep inside: I'm not really beautiful! With each passing day you fear he'll discover all the things you've done to create the outward façade of beauty, and he'll leave you.

Well, I speak to the bride in each of you now to assure you that you are unique, a thing of beauty unto God. If you'll let him, God will work in you to polish you up and present you to the world without spot or blemish! He'll be that Ephesians 3:20 God promised in His word to you. And now unto Him who *is* able to do exceeding, abundantly above all that we ask or think, according to the power that works in us (Eph. 3:20)! Be blessed by the reading of these words, in Jesus name. Amen.

Chapter I

The Anatomy Of Addiction

Addictions are powerful! Images are powerful! The most prominent image concerning you is how you look! It's the first thing they see of you when you enter a room, and many times its so powerful that it immediately defines you (first impressions): right or wrong, good or bad.

How many times have you glanced at a person of great physical beauty and hated that person instantly? Oh, no-not you! Almost without thought we begin to attribute certain <u>attri</u>butes to that person, creating distance between her and you. Or, maybe you're of that rare breed that actually desires contact with that person primarily because of their outward beauty. Congratulations, if you are of that ilk, as long as you are not seeking to lift your low self-esteem by vicarious association!

Too many of us have allowed our outward physical attributes to define us and shape our destiny, believing beauty is *all* you bring to the table. Life seems to perpetuate this myth with all the pomp and circumstance of countless beauty pageants and celebrities air brushed to perfection! So then woman, you become frantic in your efforts to measure up from early adolescence.

A simple compliment received after years of struggling with self-esteem issues, years of believing that everyone else has redeeming virtue except you, can create a whirlwind of emotions and destabilize your equilibrium. You look around and little Susie has an amazing proclivity for solving mathematical equations, Janet sings like an angel, Tammy Sue was born with a basketball in her hand

and seems to excel in every known sport—and then there stands you!

Awkward, gawky, too fat or thin, big nose or nose too tiny to breathe; you simply cannot find any redeeming value on the outside of you. No one else seems to be able to find anything either, as you seem to be the butt of every joke! Finally, one day someone sees it and gives you that first compliment: They tell you that your eyes are huge and so clear, or that you walk like royalty with your head held high and shoulders thrown back (that person did not see the pain behind the walk; an outward show of something not found within). They tell you things you only dreamed of hearing before.

Then the double whammy: you ought to be a *model*!!! How many of you have ever received that compliment? I call that compliment, the Rolls Royce of compliments: because it can impact the rest of your life.

Receiving that first significant compliment after years of suffering in the background of life can bring with it an avalanche of pain!

Okay, my secret is out. I am a recovering aging beauty! When I received the model compliment for the first time many years ago, I flipped. The little girl with the skinny legs (too skinny for the hot pants the song said make you sure of yourself), the little girl with the overlarge breasts that dwarfed her tiny body, the girl with the buck- teeth that rounded the corner before I did, had finally morphed into the similitude of a model! I became a compliment junky, a sucker for a compliment!

What heaviness descended upon me in that day of suddenly being the celebrated instead of the berated! As though I'd stepped into the bizarro world where good is bad and bad is good, and where the goat becomes the celebrated; I had arrived! I quickly picked up the phone and called Barbizon Modeling Agency in Atlanta and they sent a representative to my home to knock me off my pedestal once again. He was very polite and even made grunting noises that seemed to suggest I might have potential, but he wanted me to finish school first and then if I still felt that way about modeling, call again! Sound advice on its face, but I was suspicious of his motives. Again, feeling rejected! You're wondering if I ever realized that dream of walking some runway in Paris? The answer is no, I joined the military instead! Still, I climbed upon the roller-coaster ride of perpetual identity crisis associated with aging beauty!

Somebody is beginning to identify with what I call the entrance to the roller-coaster ride to aging beauty! In today's high fashion world 19 year- old girls are sometimes told they are too old! She begins so many times to do whatever it takes to change that person's pronouncement over her life. To those seeking beauty, the need for compliments becomes an addiction as stealthy as the devil. Like the drug addict and the alcoholic and others, I simply had to have them. I roamed the streets each day, at work or play, wondering where my next compliment would come from!

Now, before you drop this book like a hot potato screaming how dare she compare a life worshipping at the altar of beauty to the trauma of alcohol addiction or to the drug addict who must stick one more needle into his arm, read on and see that there is deliverance from all ailments no matter their name. You'll find that deliverance is found only in the man Jesus! There is help for you here no matter the name of your addiction. The bible says *every* knee shall bow and every tongue shall confess that Jesus is Lord to the glory of God! Every name that exalts itself against the knowledge of God shall be brought low! God will take you into his ample bosom, and hide you in his compassion, until you're made free from every bondage, ***including worshipping the idol god of beauty!***

There isn't much sympathy out there for aging beauties. What about the girl who has never experienced beauty at all, people ask? What about the tomboy or the girl with the long nose that only a mother could love, how about the girl with sufficient imperfections to qualify her as contestant #1 on the new television show, "The Swan?" People on this show have extensive plastic surgery, in search of the brass ring called beauty. The surgeries are so extensive that many resemble a mummy dressed for Halloween for a period of time, and suffer through intense pain and suffering to achieve what the aging beauty enjoyed for years! ***Why should they feel compassion for her when she had it all by this world's standard?***

Good question, but ***not*** one I plan to deal with in this book. For our purposes here, we agree to accept the premise that this interminable quest for beauty is an addiction worthy of its own clinic (like the Betty Ford Clinic for alcoholics). We hereby decree that aging beauties and also those in search of physical beauty exhibit behavior that is self-destructive, behavior that could lead to anorexia, bulimia, low self-esteem (leading to forms of prostitution, you don't have to be on the street to be a prostitute), and at the extreme can even lead to death! These destructive behaviors impact every area of her life as a young girl, as a wife, as a mother, and as a fulfilled woman free to do the work and the will of God! So, let's deal with this issue!

Notes

<u>Notes</u>

Chapter II

Addictions Are Power-Full

Don't let anybody tell you that your addiction to beauty is a second-class addiction! President Reagan would say, "There you go again trying to tell me I'm second class." Enough already. It's a bona-fide addiction according to Webster's definition: To give oneself up to some strong habit. *Who* will contradict the notion that extreme beauty is a lifelong habit that can consume you? We defined addiction earlier in this piece as a strong habit. Now, let's define worldly outward beauty as well, so that we have a frame of reference. This type of beauty means good looks, a very good-looking woman, ***most satisfying***.

The anatomy of addiction-active voice*!* What is the anatomy of addiction from a purely laywoman perspective? What does beauty addiction look like in terms of physical behavior? For those of you who are eggheads, how does it morph? Perhaps you look at your body excessively; for example: I used to take a mirror with me everywhere I went to make sure my make-up was right for the environment I found myself in. If the sun shines you need this amount and color, if its dark in the room then the nighttime look is better. What's in my nose? What's on my teeth (lipstick? I've rebuked that thing again and again)? Or, maybe you experience something akin to phobia about walking into a nightclub (for the unsaved) or even walking into church on Sunday morning (for the saved) without first dashing into the ladies room to check your make-up or dress!

I remember one night before I gave my life to Christ, my husband and I arrived at the Officer's Club on a base to party. While he parked the car, I dashed into the ladies room to check myself out in the mirror (mirrors are a beauty's best friend or worst nightmare!).

Everything was wrong! The wind had blown my hair with seeming hurricane force and removed all semblance of curl, and my make-up looked like day instead of night (wrong colors)! I was paralyzed with fear, I couldn't move knowing he was waiting for me outside the ladies room becoming very angry. I combed my hair that night every way possible: pinned it up, combed it down, swooped it over to one side; wiped off my make-up and put on everything in my bag of tricks. Finally, I emerged looking better, but certainly not in full bloom. Now, my husband was really angry, trying to understand, but not quite able to comprehend this fear I had of being discovered, and called out before men as a phony!

I've just introduced a new concept for scrutiny. In my case the fear of exposure as a phony beauty was overwhelming! Remember earlier I told you about the skinny young thing with big breasts and buck - teeth, she was still in there. Healing never took place inside because all my attention was diverted to the outward trying desperately to prove to people I belonged in that category. Let's face it people, I was addicted to beauty! Facing my husband that night in the club (which was just the beginning of many nights he'd wait for me to emerge from a ladies room), was very difficult because now he knew my secret. Would he use it against me? Of course not, my husband loved me, but I wasn't whole enough to comprehend that back then. If I couldn't see my way clear to receiving grace from him, you know the rest of the world terrified me!

The world can be very cruel as it practices an addiction of its own. Through the genius of television and numerous glam magazines, we've all watched entertainment programs make and break celebrities. One minute they're riding high on the covers of magazines, and the next minute they're featured on a show called, "True Hollywood Story." Because of the demands of beauty, many so-called stars lose their life to addictive behaviors: whether its through throwing up to rid the body of calories or shooting up to numb the mind to emotional pain. One minute the paparazzi whizzes about following her around Manhattan or Beverly Hills, the next minute she can't pay for publicity. As the wrinkles arrived, the offers bolted! Is it really worth your life to give yourself over to the whimsical nature of man?

Addiction knows no bounds and no reality. Addiction is not based in reality. That explains an 80 lb, 25 year-old woman's perception that she is fat and needs to diet. That explains a nicotine addict's predilection for one more cigarette over one more year of life, or the aging beauty's raging desire for one more round of plastic surgery! It seems insane, but it's real nonetheless. Addiction having no basis in reality explains much about women who give themselves over to men to pronounce pretty or ugly, good woman or bad woman, someone to keep or discard, over their life. It explains why women live so much of their lives in fear of exposure. If he's dating me because I look good, or if he married me because I look good, it naturally follows he'll leave me if I don't look good any longer. That's the ergo prompter theory: one thing necessarily leads to another. The word ergo means therefore or hence. I look bad therefore I am bad; or I look bad, therefore he's justified in finding someone else. Many of the talk shows of the 70s and the 80s corroborated this twisted belief. Thank God for God, who teaches us that marriage is a covenant relationship between two people, having nothing to do with external highs and lows!

Part of the problem is that many of you believe that man has a right to leave you when the wrinkles come and the sagging begins, despite all your best effort! Men make so many jokes about the lifespan of the woman's beauty all the time, even from the pulpit, reinforcing that a woman's place is in the beauty parlor and yes, the kitchen! This thing is so pervasive and so convincing that you don't even stop to look at your man to notice *his* pot - belly or his receding hairline! You don't even seem to notice he's not the stud *he* used to be; you only hear the plight of the aging beauty! This is a sickness same as any other addiction and we're going to break it off you today!

My heart breaks each time I hear about another woman lost to depression because of rejection due to aging. My heart breaks when a young woman is lost to anorexia or any other abuse of her body, because she's dying to be accepted and loved. I heard a news report the other day that young girls are receiving breast enhancement as a high school graduation gift! Many cited wanting to be accepted by peers as the rationale behind such radical surgery!

These young girls don't even know yet what the end will be, as they are still maturing. This urge to fit in and be acceptable to people, that drives them to such extreme behaviors, is irrational and never satisfying! Parents, instead of granting such a request for an enhanced bust, you need to recognize the request as a danger signal, deny the request, and begin to minister healing to that child!

I heard a young woman on TV say that her father never affirmed her outward beauty in any way, simply commenting that she was smart. The need to hear him say she was pretty began to consume her and the quest for beauty was on. New breasts, parents, will not heal the hurt that runs through her life, only God can do that great work. What do I recommend? Take her to church! Be the church before her eyes. Let her see your self-esteem at work.

You'd be surprised how much of this dangerous behavior of seeking validation from men all the time (or jealousy from women) has its root in the mother-daughter relationship, or in the deficit of having a father who ignores his princess and her beauty! That's one side of the coin; but, what about that same young girl when she grows up physically and becomes a ***woman***, without healing her self-esteem issues?

My soul also weeps when a women devalues herself simply because a man turns away from her to another woman to recapture his youth, or when she has to sit by and watch him ogling (to look at boldly with obvious desire) some femme fatale on the television who has been air-brushed to near perfection, had her teeth worked on spending thousands you don't have, and wearing designer clothing! My pastor once said to the men of our church: You're spending time looking at some other man's wife, clothed in finery and dripping in diamonds, and you want her over your wife; well, if she were your wife, she'd probably look and act just like your current wife. She wouldn't have fine clothes or diamonds or even a happy smile, because you're her husband now! He told the men that the countenance of their wife is a direct result of his treatment of her! (Paraphrase). That was a fine day for the women of the church!

Are you getting this girlfriend? I hope so.

Addictions are like passions, power-full!

Powerful enough to control your life and determine the direction of your future. Images feed addictions; therefore images are power-full as well, and worthy of

understanding. Let's take a deeper look at

images!

<u>Notes</u>

Notes

Chapter III

Images Are Power-Full

Actors and politicians hire image consultants because how you look to people is often more important than who you truly are inside! Can I get a witness? We have witnessed the fall of so many great men whose political image or moral image is tainted by some scandalous activity exposed. The shock is not so much that he committed the act, but more that he got caught and allowed that thing to become known. It's all so fake and phony, but it has become the hallmark of life today in the world's kingdom. At the risk of preaching, that is why you must be careful of the images that flood your mind each day. Do you want to control your message center given you by God, designed to be filled with his word alone; or are you content to let the fads and current styles of the universe dictate your personal fate? ***Images are very powerful!***

What do you imagine yourself to be? Which image stands out in your brain? When you think woman, what do you see? When you think wife, what do you see? What role does beauty play in all your musings? Answering these questions may alert you to addictive thoughts and behaviors you're harboring concerning beauty. I want to offer you a **nugget of wisdom**: Image defines you in the natural many times in a most unflattering way; but inner composure defines you in the spiritual as you really are before the God who created you in the first place. There *is* an image awaiting you, designed specifically for you by God that shapes you, and introduces you to the truth about beauty! First, you must recognize the images of the world as **only** advertising, as propaganda (widespread dissemination and/or promotion of particular ideas, doctrines and practices), and lies! Shun them!

I laugh sometimes when I think of the decades of the 70s and the 80s when my generation was coming into awareness of beauty and began to define it.

Songs played through Bose speakers at parties too numerous to remember, such as: She's a brick house; she's mighty, mighty letting it all hang out (my mind said, that's you!). Another song asked the question: Who's that lady, sexy lady, real fine lady (my mind said, that's you!)?   But there was yet another song that most of us ignored its message, "Beauty's only skin deep, yea-yea-yea; beauty's only skin deep, oh yea! I'm here to say to you today there are no truer words. ***External beauty is only skin deep! Unless you receive beauty from the Lord, it can never penetrate the skin and stay with you forever***. It can only sit upon your surface mocking you in your old age! And if you're "letting it all hang out" as a young woman, you'll have nothing later on when you need it so desperately!

Count the cost. It is an expensive proposition to consider outward beauty your only contribution to life. Don't do it. God **expands** your possibilities; it's the world that places limitations upon your head. God is the great imager! He declared through his word in Genesis 1:26, Let us make man in our own image (a moral likeness presently being formed in every believer). You truly are created in the image of God! You must see this thing through your spiritual eyes. That's what renewing the mind by the word of God is all about, **you** transformed from caterpillar to butterfly, strong and mighty because Jesus is walking out his life through you. Now you have eternal beauty; not the corruptible, aging kind of beauty men take advantage of and the world crumples beneath its feet!

God will never discard you, for he is a faithful lover! God sees your beauty because it is his! God honors your beauty because it is his! God promised in his word, "I will never leave you nor forsake you." See, this is why you need to pick up a bible quickly and learn of him, for his yoke is easy and his burden is light! You will find rest for your soul within him. God has planted a seed in someone's heart through the reading of this book (a longing for something permanent), but it needs to be watered in order to grow! You must now read the word, study and meditate upon the word, fellowship with God often (same as you have tried to fellowship with that earthly lover who rejects you), and then you must walk in what you've learned! Man may not see the God seed within you, but its still there growing inside, changing you from faith to faith and glory to glory! We're continuing the journey away from corruptible beauty, all the way to Zion!

There is nothing worse than corrupted beauty! Lucifer in the bible was an anointed cherub (one of the winged heavenly beings that support the throne of God). Lucifer was perfect, but he became lifted up with pride as illustrated in Ezekiel 28:14-17, "Thou art the anointed cherub that covers: And I have set thee so: thou wast upon the holy mountain of God; thou hast walked up and down in the midst of the stones of fire. Thou wast perfect in thy ways from the day that thou wast created, till iniquity was found in thee. By the multitude of thy merchandise they have filled the midst of thee with violence, and thou has sinned: therefore I will cast thee as profane (showing disrespect or contempt for sacred things; irreverent or blasphemous) out of the mountain of God: and I will destroy thee, O covering cherub, from the midst of the stones of fire."

Verse 17 gets to the heart of the matter, "***Thine heart was lifted up because of thy beauty,*** thou hast corrupted thy wisdom by reason of *thy* brightness: I will cast thee to the ground, I will lay thee before kings, that they may behold thee." This account in scripture of the fall of Lucifer shows us clearly the devastating effects of pride of ownership of beauty. The bible says in Proverbs 16:18: "Pride goes before destruction, and an haughty spirit before a fall." Pride lead to Lucifer, the anointed cherub's fall, and to his current fate as a laughingstock to be gazed upon by Christians in wonderment, that we ever succumbed to his phony charm or power!

Nugget of wisdom: If you are the possessor of physical beauty no matter your current chronological age, begin to give God the glory rather than yourself. After all, it is God who has done this thing, **He** has created you; you did not create yourself. That's reminiscent of giving birth to my only daughter many years ago and receiving from people compliments concerning her beauty. As is the custom, I always said thank you as though somehow I was responsible for creating that beauty. Give God today a holy and vigorous "pat on the back" for creating you in a manner that is good, and you'll immediately begin changing your atmosphere from one of conceit and deceit, to one of praise and thanksgiving! Don't exalt that gift from God higher in your life than the Creator himself, *that's* profane!

When you begin to see outward beauty in its proper context, you will truly experience a paradigm shift! Suddenly, in the deepest recesses of your belly, you'll know that God is the author of all beauty, and you will then break forth in spontaneous praise and thanksgiving. The praise and thanksgiving makes you like a farmer. Did you ever think you'd want to be a farmer? A farmer sows seed and receives a harvest in kind.

When you sow praise and thanksgiving unto God, there is a shift that will take place in your atmosphere. Your focus becomes who he is to you, rather than who you are to you. Your harvest will be in kind as you'll begin to know intimately who you are in him! Someone has referred to this new relationship as an exchange of who(s)! You tell God who he is to you, and he shows you who you are to him. This is amazing because once you know how God sees you, you'll be able to put behind you man's lopsided assessment of you. Freedom at last!

As you remain on this journey from depression or uncertainty to joy in Jesus, you'll fulfill scripture! Look at you. God will use you to fulfill scripture! That simple fact alone raises you from the doldrums of believing you're only as good as your face is pretty, all the way to hallelujah anyhow! I'm getting excited for you! Psalm 100 expresses this best, "Make a joyful noise unto the Lord, all ye lands. Serve the Lord with gladness: Come before his presence with singing (Heb. means to shout (for joy) or to rejoice)."

Whether you can carry a tune or not, you *can* shout for joy, you can rejoice before the Lord to fulfill this scripture! "Know ye that the Lord he is God: it is he that hath made us and not we ourselves (told ya); we are his people, and the sheep of his pasture." What a revelation! You can change your reality and your daily atmosphere through praise and worship of your creator, God! Then God in turn will tell you the truth about yourself. What is this truth?

Beloved, you haven't heard a compliment until you hear one from the mouth of God. God will tell you that you are more than that new dress from Saks 5th Avenue or Wal-Mart (no matter)! God will tell you emphatically that you are his chosen one. The Great I Am, the Creator of the Universe, the God who is more than enough, will whisper to your heart that you are chosen by him to bear fruit and that your fruit shall be of the lasting variety (not birthed in pettiness!). God will tell you that you are fearfully and wonderfully made, no matter what those around you may say. Arise, go look in the real mirror (the Word of God) and for the first time ever see yourself beyond the horizon of littleness! Jump for joy, child of God, for you look marvelous: how do you do it? The answer is emphatically: ***by the power of God!***

<u>Notes</u>

Notes

Chapter IV

Be Ye Transformed By Renewing Your Mind

Hopefully you saw this chapter coming long before now. Hopefully you discerned the need through our discussions for transformation by the word of God. If you're ever going to accept that beauty comes from within, your thinking must transcend the myths this world actively and vigorously perpetuates.

Romans 12:2 emphatically states, "And be not conformed (shaped and molded) to this world: but be ye transformed (the Gr. Word is Metamorphoo meaning transfigured, or having your outward changed by a supernatural move of God, so as to exalt or glorify) by the renewing of your mind, that you may prove what is that good, and acceptable, and perfect, will of God."

Let's take a brief look at the great transfiguration of Jesus on the Mount of Transfiguration. Chapter 17 of Matthew speaks of this outward change of Jesus, which stunned three of his disciples. Verses 1-2, "And after six days Jesus takes Peter, James, and John his brother, and bringeth them up into an high mountain apart, and was transfigured before them: and his face did shine as the sun, and his raiment was white as the light." You're not impressed right? Jesus was after all the Son of God, not a mere mortal like you! Moses in Exodus 34:29-35 was transfigured! "And it came to pass, when Moses came down from mount Sinai with the two tables of testimony in Moses' hand, when he came down from the mount, that Moses wist (Heb yada meaning to know) not that the skin of his face shone while he talked with him." Moses was transfigured! His face shone to the degree that he put a veil on his face until he finished speaking with the people!

You're still not impressed, right? Jesus was the Son of God, Moses was in Old Testament days; this is a new day! Well, Stephen in the New Testament (Acts 6:15) was also transfigured. Stephen was on trial for his life, brought up before the council and accused by false witnesses of speaking blasphemous words against the holy place and against the law of that day. Verse 15, "And all that sat in the council, looking steadfastly on him, saw his face as it had been the face of an angel."

That was God's glory shining through the face of Stephen supernaturally, to convince the people of the truth of his words! Are you convinced now beloved that through constant fellowship with the Holy Ghost, you too can be transfigured before men? Your face can begin to shine with the light of God's truth! Men and women will be set free and delivered as they see the light of God shining forth through you, and because you spoke God's word over their circumstances!

I present to you true beauty: ***<u>the glory of God shining forth through you daily!</u>*** I believe this is one book that delivers. You do not need yet another image consultant! You do not need one more compliment! ***You simply need God!*** The God of Jesus Christ, who will give you the Holy Spirit as the earnest of your eternal inheritance of beauty! I'll leave you with one last scriptural secret from God found in 1 Chronicles 16: 29, "Give unto the LORD the glory due unto his name: bring an offering, and come before him: worship the LORD in the beauty of holiness." Together, we've discovered the true definition of beauty (drum-roll please!): ***<u>its holiness</u>!*** Holiness makes you irresistible to God *and* man!!!

Now, go be beautiful! God bless you, amen!

<u>Notes</u>

Notes

-*Prayer of Confession*-

Father, I come to you in the name of Jesus. I confess with my mouth that I am a sinner. I ask you to forgive my sins and come into my heart as my Lord and Savior. I am turning my life over to you! Jesus, fill me with your Holy Spirit and make me who you would have me to be. I believe I am now saved, and will serve you for the rest of my life! In Jesus name I pray, amen.

Please sign below and mail this page to me so that I can be in prayer for your growth and development in Christ! Be sure to find a church home where the full Bible is taught and lived!

Today, _____
                              Date

I, _____
                      Your name

I've accepted Jesus Christ as my Lord and
Savior. My mailing address is (optional):

_____

_____

_____

E-Mail to: Evangelist C. K. Inniss

cynmar_enterprises@juno.com

PERFECT SEVEN

We can celebrate each day of our life in Christ Jesus as though it's special. The Bible teaches us in Romans 12:2, to be transformed by the renewing of our mind! Here is a plan for soul renewal and prosperity! Each week is the week of weeks! Seven days of perfection when you name your days:

Miracle Monday (atmosphere of expectancy; practicing looking up for miracles)!

Tangible Touch Tuesday (expecting a personal touch of God's Holy Power)!

Wisdom Wednesday (delving into the Word with The Teacher, Blessed Holy Spirit)!

Trinity Thursday (doing at least one holy action for the Father, one holy action for the Son, and one holy action for the Holy Ghost)!

Freedom Friday (whom the Son sets free is free indeed; enjoying this day as the end of your work week, or simply as a day of focusing on the freedom Jesus died to secure for you)!

Saturation Saturday (receiving and basking in a heavy dose of the anointing)!

Soothing Sunday (day of rest, what is more restful than praising God?)!

Any one of these things can occur on any day and/or every day; but on that specific day, focus on the specified area!

<u>Notes</u>

Notes

To purchase copies of "God Still Loves Aging Beauties" contact Feast of the Lord Ministries at:
http://www.lulu.com/cynthiainniss

Dr. C.K. Inniss

cynmar_enterprises@juno.com

Cover design by Marco A. Inniss of cynmar-t-designs

<u>OTHER WORKS BY AUTHOR</u>
<u>COMING SOON</u>

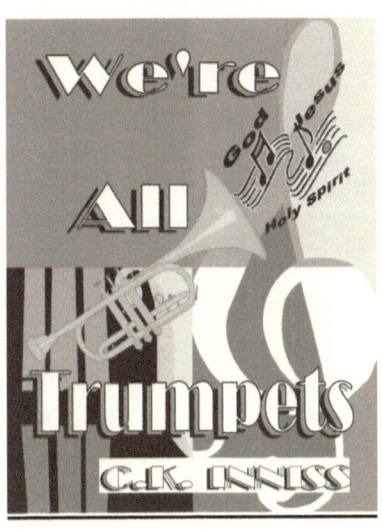

We're All Trumpets

C.K. Inniss

Your life will become the evidence that you are God's Holy Ghost filled, fire baptized trumpeter of the gospel of Jesus Christ, and of His Word. Once you've read this book and digested the body of evidence therein, you'll begin to image yourself as a trumpet, or at the very least a trumpeter, heralding: The gospel of Jesus Christ, the Kingdom of God which **is** at hand, and trumpeting the soon return of our Lord. The sounds you make while trumpeting will bring teaching, preaching, and healing to a lost and dying world, same as Jesus did. (Matt. 4:23)

OTHER WORKS BY AUTHOR
COMING SOON

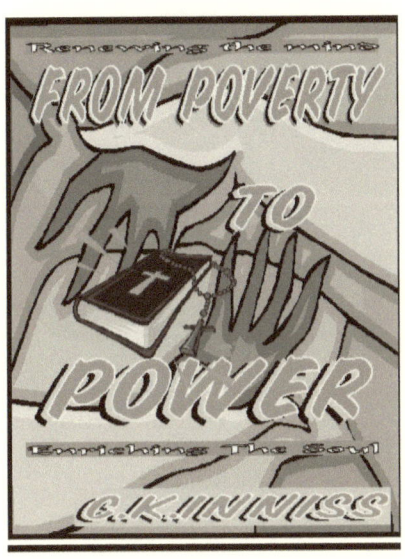

From Poverty To Power

C.K. Inniss

This work is simply intended to expound upon scripture, not replace it! " From Poverty to Power" will help to illuminate the condition of your soul, thereby paving the way for God's promised prosperity to flood your soul and change your life!